Hit by a Brick

by

Deborah D Johnson

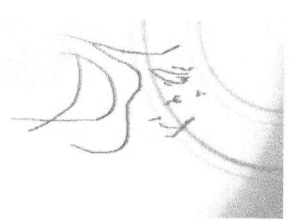

ISBN: **1518733476**
ISBN-13: **978-1518733475**

DEDICATION

To my loving family and friends who continue to encourage me to write and share my experiences that will help others find the joy and strength in all of life's challenges.

CONTENTS

FOREWORD

This is a true story. I will not share the actual names and places where this occurred. There is some amusement in this writing. But there are also some details that are not appropriate for all readers. This book may not be appropriate for those who are sensitive to discussions about the body or who are too young to understand the context.

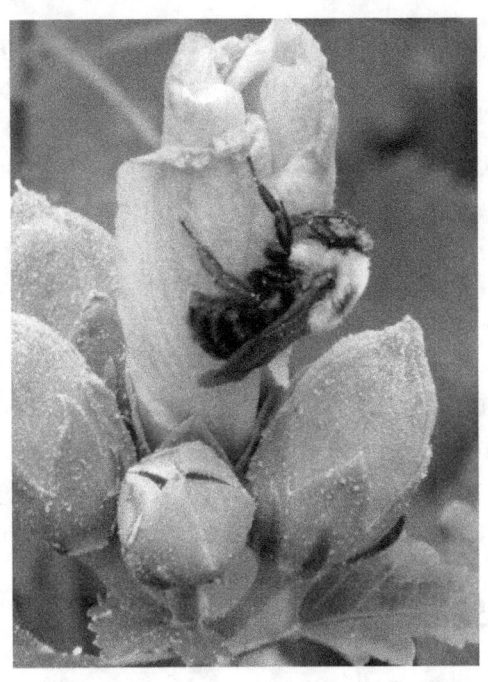

CHAPTER 1 INTERRUPTION OF MY SCHEDULE

I'm a regular person going about my retirement (but not really) days. Unforeseen by me, I have established a hectic schedule. Not on purpose, mind you. At least I don't think so.

Well, I'm writing, volunteering, running a publishing company. I'm long on dreams, vision, energy. But really short on funds. So, add to this schedule, the stress of trying to find the funds to pay for it.

Oh yes, I can pay my share of household bills with my "good government" retirement check. At least until heating, electricity and food costs started climbing. I still make out fine. I simply can't do some things I used to do. What were those? Unimportant. Suffice it to say, I am okay with what I had to cut out.

I need to get back to my level of tithing I'm accustomed to. Supporting my church is important to me and I have not been as supportive, monetarily, lately. Oh I still volunteer my time so I give physical support. I teach Sunday School and sing in a choir. Blah, blah, blah...

Well, I also walking regularly and go to a local fitness center to Zumba once or twice a week.

Now what's this cancer thing?

So, as you can see, life's really not bad for me. I'm doing fine. Doing my thing and still keeping the house clean, I think. I also still prepare breakfast, lunch, snack and a pretty good dinner almost daily for my hubby. Sounds like a super person right?

It sounds like a crazy person or simply a workaholic as I've sometimes been called.

Looking at my schedule, you might ask, where's the fun. Writing is fun for me. Well, until I became a professional and published author.

Zumba was fun until I stopped suddenly. Why did I stop? I had sort of an interruption of my schedule. I said "my schedule" so maybe it wasn't God's schedule.

Where shall I start? How about right here.

Now what's this cancer thing?

Yes, the "C" word. Actually the big "C" word. Big "C" to me anyway.

I got my phone call as many others have before me, and many others will after.

Wow, what a shocker. A doctor calls to give me test results. You probably know this story. It's not so unusual. I had my annual mammogram. I received a call from a doctor indicating something was found and that more tests were necessary.

Good doctors go above and beyond what's okay to reach you to give you troubling test results. I know this because a long time ago, I received a call from a doctor on a Sunday evening. This time, the doctor called me multiple times; leaving messages on our home phone and my cell. We were out of town enjoying a brief break. As soon as I could, I called back.

Then I got the word.

Doctors don't necessarily say they found something that may be cancer or cancerous over the phone. Maybe they think we will pass out or do something really stupid. This one said something like "according to the test results we found "_____" fill in the blank with the name of the type of cancer.

Then there was this pause as I digested the information. Then I asked the obvious question. What does that mean? Then another pause, then the doctor got pretty close to the "C" word like carcinoma _____ something or other. Think about it. This conversation can't be fun for the doctor either, at least a good and caring doctor.

Anyway, let me continue.

Another pause as I think some more. Then I say "Carcinoma sounds like cancer." The doctor indicates that that sounds about right.

Another pause as I try to think of something to

say. Finally it comes.

"Well Dr. _____, what's next?" Then the real conversation began.

PAY BACK

I've been responsible most of my life.

Worked so long I don't remember not working.

I did jobs that I hated and loved but worked hard in all of them.

Ask anyone who knows me.

Now I believe it is time for a return on my life long investment.

What investment?

- Hard working
- Reliable
- Kind (I think)
- Long suffering (really long)
- Forgiving
- Smiling even when mistreated or forgotten or left out (on purpose)

You know. That Christianity stuff.

I have believed in God so long I don't remember when I didn't.

Sometimes I feel like David in asking God, How long must I suffer?

How long must I wait?

How long…

I don't know.

God knows.

*"Pride goeth before destruction, and a haughty spirit
before a fall."*

Proverbs 16:18 KJV

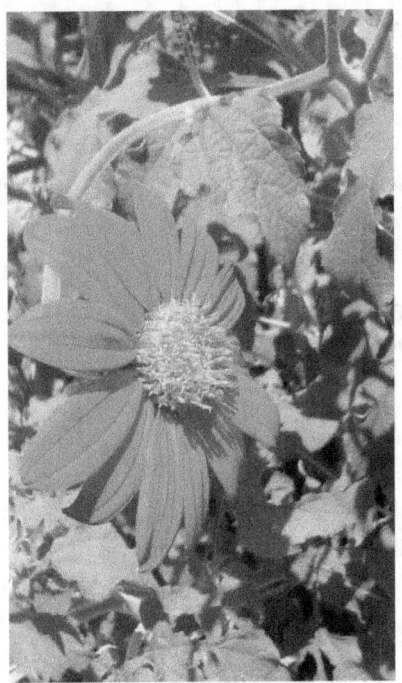

CHAPTER 2 A BRIEF PAUSE

I'll pause for a moment here and talk just a bit about my biopsy experience. Here are the steps the first set of doctors took along the road to determine if I really had something. At this point my mammogram showed something unusual.

After my annual diagnostic mammogram, the doctors found something different from my last one. They told me right away that I needed to have a biopsy (#1). I had one of these before a few years ago, so I basically knew what to expect. I scheduled the appointment.

If you have not had one of these before, I will provide some details. If you have, then just skip this part and go to the next section. However you may want to spend a couple of minutes on memory lane just to see if your experience matched mine or was totally different.

For breast biopsies, I was placed face down on a table with two holes in it. My breasts were placed into those holes. You need to be pretty trusting to do this. Then the "crew" raises the table so they can get under me. Here's where it gets interesting. I feel someone fooling around with my breasts, but I can't see what they are doing.

> If you have a good doctor he/she will talk to you throughout this process…

They squeeze the appropriate one in some sort of clamping device and take x-rays to find the exact spot where the biopsy should be taken. This took a while. The second one didn't take nearly as long (#2). Yes I had to go through this a second time; same breast different location.

When the "crew" thought they had my breast in the right position in came Doctor _____. She said hello to me then dropped under the table with the "crew". Here's where the fun really started. I'm told not to move throughout the entire procedure and now that my breast was clamped into position, I really didn't want to move no matter what.

You know what's coming next. Yep, they have to numb me. How in the world do they expect you not to move with your breast twisted in a clamp which you cannot see and they stick you with something that you also cannot see.

But… I was happy for the numbing stuff. I wouldn't want to go through this procedure without it.

Okay, you guessed it. I was the good smiling patient, I think, and I didn't move so we're off to a great start.

If you have a good doctor he/she will talk to you throughout this process particularly since they know you are awake and can't see what they are doing. They also want to make sure you don't suddenly jump if they do something unexpected.

The doctor told me what she was doing.
Cutting at the best spot to take the tissue
sample. I felt the instrument but felt no pain.
Yippee! The doctor continued talking and told
me when she found the spot. She said
something like this, "Ms. Johnson, I am taking
the biopsy now. You're doing great. Please
don't move." (By the way, if you move they
have to start all over again. Oh no. Not with me
they won't!)

So yes, I kept still. It was hard but doable. No
pain. I'm okay. Just way ready to get up off
that table and get my breasts out of those
holes.

The doctor continued speaking to me. "Okay, I
have the tissue. Please continue to not move
because now I have to leave for a few minutes
and check if this is the sample from the right
place. She left.

If you have a good "crew', they will talk to you
to keep you calm and completely still while
waiting for the doctor to return. Mine did.
Someone even rubbed my back a bit. It was
soothing. I couldn't talk to them but they talked
to me.

The doctor returned and said she had the right
sample from the right place. I breathed a sigh

of relief as the clamp came off and I was allowed to sit up. Oh no, it's not over yet. One member of the "crew' patched me up and gave me care instructions with an ice pack and bandages.

Someone else entered the room and told me that the biopsy was inconclusive and another one must be taken. I was too shaky to fully consider this at the time. I made another appointment for biopsy number 2 and went home to wait.

To make a long story short, I had the second biopsy in a couple of weeks after the first one. Not fully healed. Yes, that one found the spot and it became official that I needed to see a surgeon.

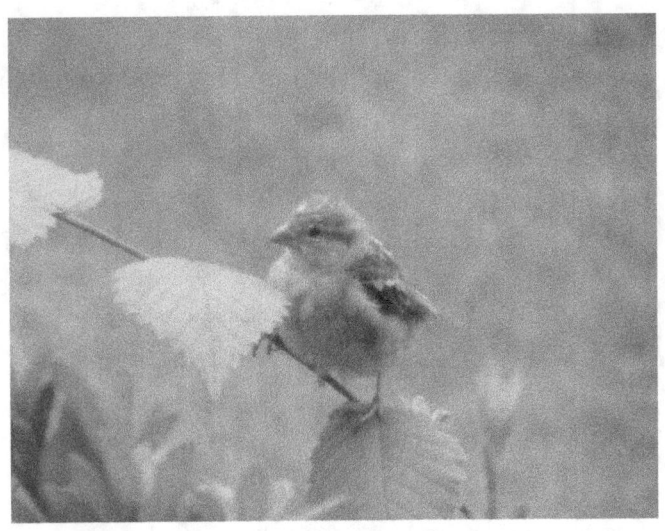

CHAPTER 3 WHAT'S NEXT?

I later received a call and was given a short list of recommendations for doctors and cancer centers that accepted my insurance. Writing rapidly, I tried to keep my mind blank. I was home alone at the time.

I hung up, picked a hospital that my husband and I liked. I made the call. I got my first appointment and was on my way. To what, I didn't really know.

How about erasing this cancer thing from my body? Not happening.

But I needed movement to something. Hopefully getting this stuff out of my body!

Then I picked up the phone and called my husband. Later we told our children then a few friends. Prayers started going up for me. I could feel the love and support.

Thank God for insurance even though it is expensive. My list of doctors would have been pretty empty without it. I probably would not have had the mammogram and two biopsies that found the cancer in the first place if I didn't have insurance.

First appointment went extraordinarily well. Staff was polite and supportive. Doctor was friendly. She listened to me and answered my questions in a way I could understand. What more could I ask for? How about erasing this cancer thing from my body? Not happening.

We set the plan and schedule. The tests began. Another mammogram, an MRI and another biopsy. Okay, I just had two not that long ago. Another one?

But guess what? Testing did not end easily. Some interesting results came from my third biopsy (#3). Yep, had to have another one (#4); an MRI biopsy. This was just in case there was no more cancer than they first thought. I am sick of biopsies. But wait, I do still have appropriate health insurance to have an MRI biopsy. I should not complain too much. Although, I am really tired and really, *really* sore about now.

The MRI biopsy was even more interesting than the others. Different place. Same doctor as the last one, so I'm happy. Similar process as the second one, only once I was placed on a table with the holes, I was pushed gently into the MRI tube. I was happy for once to be face down on my stomach with my head on a soft pillow.

I could not see anything. I heard voices telling me what was going on and reminding me not to move. All the while I listened to my favorite music through head phones during breaks in the conversation. I'm not talking. They are. Remember I couldn't move. I did have a panic button. Music and panic button worked for me.

I really had to concentrate on the music and breathe real slow, but softly. I didn't want them to have to start over again. I really wanted to go running and screaming out of the tube, around the room and out of the room. Then, continue my hollering all the way to get my clothes and run away.

What a picture. A grown up screaming down the hallway in a hospital gown. This was a nice thought but I didn't do it. First of all, I knew I needed this fourth biopsy so the surgeon and her team would know precisely what I had and the appropriate method to remove what they found.

Ultimately, I kept still. God only knows how. It was hard at times. I really didn't want to do this again. I had to hold on so I prayed and sang in my head. No moving. I made it through my final biopsy. Once it was over, I was shaky all over. I think I hid this very well though. At least I tried to. When the doctor said it was over, I tried real hard not to just leap off the table and run as I described before.

They had to remove the IV after all. Oh did I say that I did get an IV inserted in my arm so some ink/die stuff could be shot in my body to highlight the questionable area in my breast? IV's are usually no fun either. But the entire team was kind, patient and efficient with me.

Okay celebration moment. There was no additional cancer other than what they first found. My doctor was finally sure about how to proceed. Whoop! Whoop!

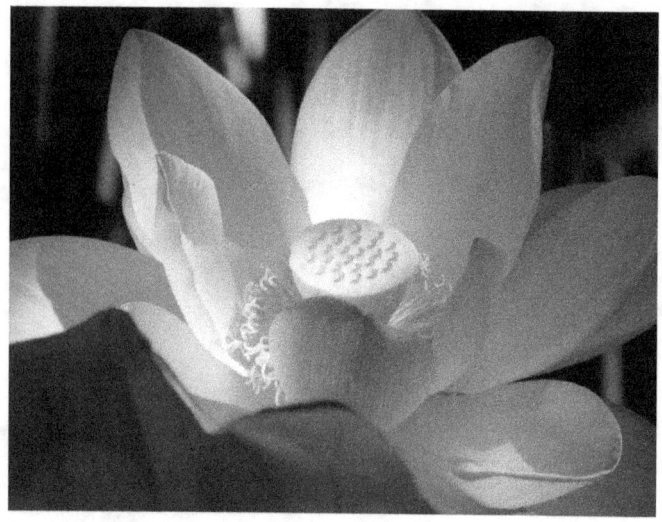

Chapter 4 My Diagnosis

Done again. Patched up again and sent home. The tests went well. The surgeon showed me the test results and gave me her diagnosis - Ductal Carcinoma in Situ (DCIS). She then explained her strategy for me. I would have surgery, a lumpectomy with lymph node biopsy followed immediately by Interoperative Radiation Therapy (IORT).

I had to see a radiologist to confirm the strategy. Off I go. I hope you are not bored yet because this is where things get really interesting, but not in a bad way. God put me in the hands of excellent doctors and techies in an awesome place.

Have you ever had a doctor who was a comedian? My radiologist was one. It worked for me. What I didn't need at this serious time was to meet with a somber and serious doctor.

The radiologist was surprising. He made me laugh. He lightened me up for a moment in what looked like a life threatening situation. And I didn't want to die. The serious stuff was mixed in with the light-heartedness. He examined me as he joked with me. He reviewed my test results with me and my husband. I relaxed enough to listen, ask questions and take notes.

> I like to talk about everything, I'm told, and I probably do.

He said that my doctor's recommendations seemed to be the appropriate approach and that he would follow up with her. I like when doctors who are treating me talk to each other. Makes me feel so much better. We left and moved on with the rest our day.

Next came the wait for surgery. Here is where the whole family cheers you on or wants to talk about it or not talk about it at all. I had the combination. Family stopped by that I hadn't seen in quite some time.

I like to talk about everything, I'm told, and I probably do. I need to dump stuff out of my head to a sounding board, a good listener. Since so many people have gone through what I was going through, it was, and still is, hard to find someone who will just sit and listen.

Even before I finish my statement, there are those who jump in and say "I have a friend, relative... going through the same thing. They are stage_____. The doctors found yours early so you should be fine." I smile even though I haven't been allowed to finish my statement. I understand that what they say is true.

However, I'm in a situation I don't want to be in although it isn't unto death so I feel the need to be heard. I also feel small because so many others are in way worse situations than my own. I move on.

Looking at the calendar, I await the date to go to the hospital.

I am fairly internet capable. While I waited for surgery, I searched the web for information on my diagnosis. I wanted as much information about my situation that I could find. After all, I have heard the "C" word and I still don't get the difference between a little "c" and a big "C".

For me, it's just big "C" and I need to have surgery and some form of radiation treatment. I couldn't talk as much as I wanted about my feelings so I went into a frenzy of information gathering. Reading all I could find to settle my mind. The waiting was hard.

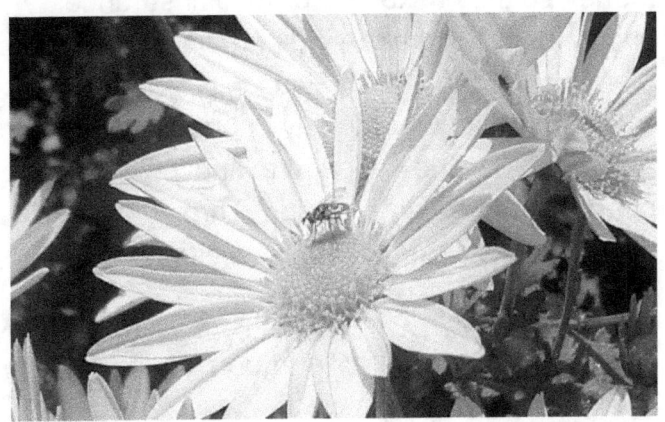

CHAPTER 5 SURGERY AND FOLLOW UP

Surgery day arrived. It's in and out so I selected and donned my most relaxed-fit outfit. I made sure I didn't eat or drink after a certain time the day before and placed my insurance card, credit/debit card and ID in my bag as the hospital requires these items at check in.

One of my best friends insisted on meeting us at the hospital. I was touched. Maybe someone actually noticed my shaking visage and "deer in the headlights" stare and understood that I needed a little extra hand holding.

Hospital check-in went smoothly. Everyone I

met was polite and friendly. They wanted their money so they asked for proof of insurance and payment of the fee. My husband handed them his card for which I was very grateful. I was still shaking, not visibly I hoped. I passed along my ID. They needed to know they were operating on the right person. Throughout the day, I was asked to identify myself. I guess it is best to be safe than sued.

Since I had an excellent surgeon, I knew what to expect on surgery day. I would be checked in. Then, I would be sent off for a couple of pre-surgery procedures.

> If you have had surgery before, raise your hand.

I changed into hospital attire and was given a fluffy robe to wear. Awesome. It was nice and soft, big enough to cover me completely so I am warm and comfortable. Settled into a cushioned high backed chair. I'm happy they had me sitting up and not lying down on a hospital bed.

Then I had the IV needle inserted into my hand by a wonderful techie. He numbed the spot first so I didn't feel a thing as he slid that huge needle into place. Awesome again. I had two other stops before surgery.

Off we go as I'm wheeled around the hospital by other nice techie people to my pre-surgery process locations. I smiled and made jokes along the way. I waved at passersby like I was some wealthy heiress or queen. All who I came across smiled back and humored me. I actually wanted to lighten up a difficult situation for the good of the people who were taking care of me. I hope it worked. It helped me lighten up at least.

I was taken to the techies who were charged with finding the location for the surgery. The techies then placed a wire in me, ultimately, to point the surgeon to the right spot. I also went to the techies who inserted a die in me so that the surgeon could see what to look for. I am simplifying the process here but this is basically what happened.

All stuff pointing to the right place, I'm ready for surgery. By the way, everybody who came to me to check something or do something initialed my left side where the surgery would be performed. After a while I had quite a few initials on me. I had my husband take a picture. No I am not including it here.

If you have had surgery before, raise your

hand. Probably a lot of you have. The very idea of handing over my body to someone who I thought was trustworthy and capable was daunting. I had to go to sleep and wake up all fixed and happy, in faith. Okay, that was doable. I already knew God had placed me in excellent hands.

I was taken to the operating room where all these people were hustling and bustling about. They were waiting and preparing for me!

As I said before, it helps when people really talk to you—tell you what they are doing and what they are about to do. As they were talking, I was moved about, adjusted, connected to devices. We cracked a few jokes then I went into the dark.

When I woke, the first person I saw was my doctor. She was smiling. Nice to see her smile. She told me that all went well and they got everything, including removing some lymph nodes. My husband and friend came in to see me. I was so happy to see them. It is good to have a loved one or two to look at once waking up from surgery.

This was my second major surgery in three years. The previous one, I stayed in the hospital for a few days. This one, they sent me right home with good drugs. I was happy to go right home and even happier about the strange but comfortable bra they put on me, the ice packs and good drugs. All necessary for a comfortable recovery.

Yes, I did have radiation treatment, but it was done directly on the affected site in my breast right after surgery. As planned.

Before I went home, I did have to return that nice fluffy robe and put on my own clothes. It was a nice robe.

I must say that I have the most excellent friends. I really don't know how this happened because I don't believe I have been a good friend to them. Somehow they have hung with me anyway.

My husband needed to return to work. I had follow up on appointments to go through.

One day, I received a phone call from one friend who was not happy with me. I've been keeping everybody informed on my healing progress and appointments. She asked why I did not ask her to take me to my appointments. I don't know why I was surprised.

First I was stunned then shamed. I thought to

myself, *why hadn't I asked anyone to help.* Did this mean I have no faith in my friends? Did this mean that I am too independent? Maybe I am too proud. To this day, I am not sure. I just felt stupid at the time, but grateful. Very, very grateful.

My friend drove me to my first follow up appointment. I don't know about you but I was not looking forward to going to another "cancer institute". My previous major surgery was done by a doctor in a "cancer institute".

This was a bit too much for me. It was good to have company. I didn't realize how weak I was after surgery until I had to walk from her car, through the lobby and to the doctor's office. I needed to sit in the lobby for a few minutes to rest. Luckily, we arrived for my appointment early. Also just a luckily, someone was singing in the lobby. We listened to the melodious and soothing voice accompanied by someone playing a grand piano. Nice.

I got my breath back, stood and leaned on my friend as we continued our progress.

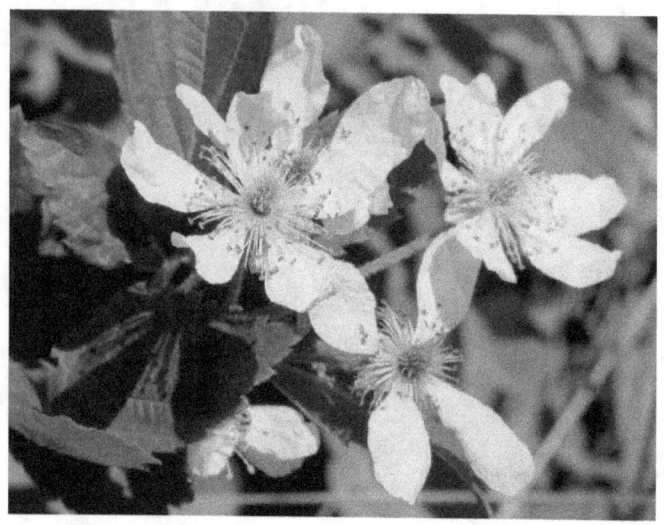

CHAPTER 6 BACK TO MY SCHEDULE?

I had the surgery as originally planned with radiation treatment directly on the spot where the cancer was found. No more radiation treatment was necessary. No chemotherapy was necessary. Good news right?

Yes, most definitely. Back to my schedule?

Not just yet.

I had to make an appointment to see an oncologist. Didn't really know why I needed to see an oncologist or else I wasn't listening anymore to my surgeon after she told me all the cancer was removed. Didn't want to listen anymore. I didn't want to see an oncologist. My family and friends insisted so I agreed.

I was still in pain one month later. I don't think anyone believed me. I felt pain and burning while sitting in meetings or working from home. Taking drugs every day is not an option for me. I was told to take what I needed to feel better.

Oh boy. I believe that God has healed me from cancer even though I'm still not sure why he allowed it in the first place. I'm human. I have doubts, hopes and fears. All this plays on all of the above. Where do I take my stand?

Inside, I am kicking and screaming like a spoiled child.

I am getting back to some semblance of normal life. But what's normal after a cancer diagnosis?

Anyway, I started scheduling meetings for the second Civil Service book, writing my sections, researching, when needed. My oncologist appointment was coming. I started my list of questions as my friends advised. I purposed in myself to have my questions. Make the doctor take time to listen to me and talk to me. She did. She is an excellent doctor too. She actually started out by giving me a big smile and an even bigger hug.

I was not easily going to get away from my doctors. For the next five years, I am to take Arimidex (Anastrozole) along with a few vitamins and visit the cancer institute every 3 months or so for checkups to be sure the cancer does not return. My schedule is not my own just yet.

Inside, I am kicking and screaming like a spoiled child. They got everything, right? Why do I need to continue to see a cancer doctor in a cancer institute? I'm healed right?

As I said before, my radiologist has an excellent sense of humor. At my follow up appointment with him, he was both happy and serious. He was happy the surgery turned out so well and that I only needed one radiation treatment. He said he's had to tell other patients something different; that they needed additional radiation treatments. He was happy he didn't have to say this to me.

Then he went all serious on me. He turned on his serious face (hadn't seen this one before) as he explained to me why I needed to see an oncologist and go through this 5-year process. He wanted to make sure he did not see me again under worse circumstances. He usually smiled a lot but not this time. I got the message.

The oncologist handles the preventative stuff. Okay, Okay I got it. Didn't like it, but I got it. I can be and still am pretty stubborn at times.

Now back to my busy schedule? Not quite yet. Researching things that I am not supposed to eat. Changing my diet. No small task. Trying to take pills every day. This is a first for me. Several months later and I still haven't gotten back to my schedule. Lots of crazy stuff going on in the world. I can't get too busy again. But I need to be involved somehow.

Yes, I asked God many times why he allowed me to have this cancer thing. I'm still waiting for His answer. Right now I'm thinking maybe it was to interrupt my busy schedule.

A friend of mine is telling me that I am becoming a bit grouchy. A first for me, I hope. My life has been disrupted by something tough, so she called me on my attitude. But she understands.

"And we know that all things work together for good to those who love God, to those who are the called according to His purpose."

Romans 8:28 New King James Version (NKJV)

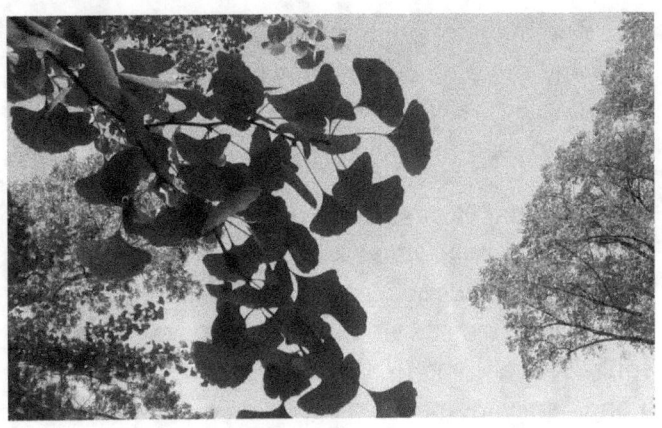

CHAPTER 7 DUCTAL CARCINOMA IN SITU (DCIS)

When I was diagnosed with DCIS, the first question I asked was "What does that mean?" Well, I needed a plain English definition. As any other red blooded fairly proficient web surfer would do, I went online.

> Ductal carcinoma in situ (DCIS) is the presence of abnormal cells inside a milk duct in the breast. DCIS is considered the earliest form of breast cancer.
>
> DCIS is noninvasive, meaning it hasn't spread out of the milk duct to invade other parts of the breast.
> mayoclinic.org
> (accessed Sept 21, 2015)

I am not much for printing out stuff so I had to go back and recreate some of my research for you. There was much information on this, but I first wanted to read the sights I thought most reputable.

The **National Breast Cancer Foundation, Inc**. contains a helpful video with an easily understood explanation of what Ductal Carcinoma in Situ (DCIS) is. This site would be a great start when you're researching to understand you or your friend/family member's diagnosis.

There are more complex sources of information. More detailed information along with symptoms can be found here at **Breast Cancer.org**.

As your research continues, I advise staying away from those sites whose primary/obvious business is advertising their services or product. It is important now to get accurate information. Accuracy will lead to better decisions and less fear. I do believe knowing is much better than guessing.

Other sites to check out:

Mayo Clinic.org

My Cancer Treatment.org

Whatever the diagnosis, we are to take an active role in our treatment. From the start. Know what is happening to you (diagnosis), what will happen/the plan (treatment), and what happens next (future treatments/medications). Also know the risks at each of these stages.

The diagnosis of cancer is scary enough. At least it was for me. Know the real story. Having real and clear information

> Fear cannot keep us from action.

helped me get past that fear. Getting past the fear got me to treatment much easier.

When I learned that DCIS is a very early stage of cancer and is treatable, I was happy but still scared. The fear did not and has not gone away, but it is manageable. Any cancer diagnosis can engender all kinds of imaginings in our human selves. This should be expected and acknowledged.

Fear cannot keep us from action.

I thank God that this one for me was not as bad as I imagined. For me, there are things I can do to take charge of my health and my treatment.

Have a mammogram

I now am a chief advocate for regularly scheduled mammograms. I don't like them. Yes, they are uncomfortable. My cancer was only detectable through mammograms followed by biopsies.

I have diagnostic mammograms which basically means that more X-rays are taken than with a screening mammograms and I am told immediately the results. I don't have to wait a few days to get something in the mail.

I had a biopsy a few years ago in which the results came back benign. Since that time, I have had diagnostic mammograms. In addition, I pay for the 3D mammogram which is supposed to be even more accurate.

My insurance did not cover this kind of mammogram so I had to pay for it. Not all places that give mammograms offer the 3D version.

Ultimately, talk to your doctor about when you should have mammograms and about what kind is appropriate for you. Mammograms save lives.

"A scorner seeketh wisdom, and findeth it not: but knowledge is easy unto him that understandeth."

Proverbs 14:6 KJV

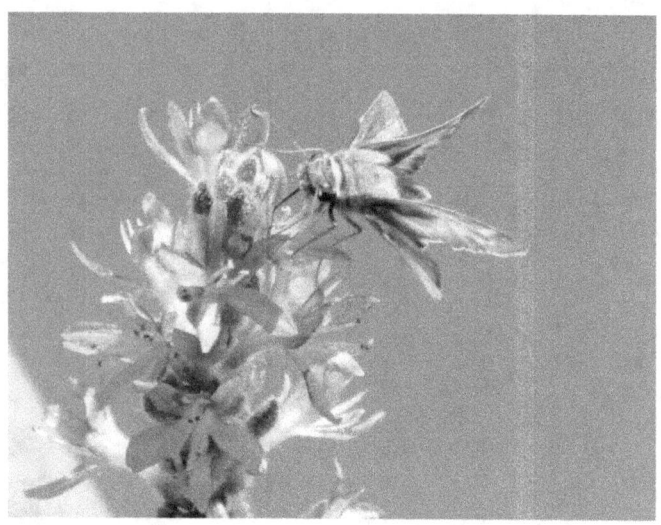

CHAPTER 8 ME AND SOY PRODUCTS

I was told that my body make up is sensitive to soy products. Therefore I should avoid soy products. Before I was diagnosed, I took a daily supplement of a soy product to help reduce the symptoms of menopause. I immediately stopped taking this product.

From that time, I have tried to moderate or eliminate soy products in my diet. Let me tell you. It is almost impossible to completely eliminate soy products from your diet. Soy in some form seems to be in nearly everything, from breads to nonstick low fat cooking spray. Most items that indicate they contain vegetable oil means soybean oil.

This is a tough road. Research is inconclusive on the effect of soy on breast cancer. What to do has been confusing. Right now I go by what my doctor said. In my case, minimize soy intake.

This is a daily challenge. I have started reading the most finest of fine print on products to determine soy content. I

> Moderation is the key in most things.

have found that even products that contain no soy may contain soy because they were prepared in facilities that produce soy products.

I never liked tofu so that is not a problem for me. I love what traditionally is called "Chinese Food" which contains soy. I also love Thai food. My dilemma has been on how much soy is too much.

Well. I really try to not call a lot of attention to myself when I go out to lunch, dinner, breakfast with others about this but sometimes I have to, especially when we end up in a Thai restaurant.

Because I was told this does not mean that this would be the appropriate approach for you.

Here's some information on the research to date on soy and breast cancer. The results are inconsistent.

- **Breast Cancer.org: Soy Research**
- **Cancer Center Treatments of America: Nuts about soy?**
- **Breast Cancer.org: Eating soy…**

Okay. So what do you do now? Check with your doctor. See a nutritionist about what works and does not work for you. Soy seems to affect people in different ways. Some in good ways and some in not so good ways. At this point, no one can tell for sure but the research continues.

I have found that I should moderate what I eat no matter what. Too much of anything is not good for me and probably not for you.

Moderation is the key in most things.

"So, whether you eat or drink, or whatever you do, do all to the glory of God."

1 Corinthians 10:31 (ESV)

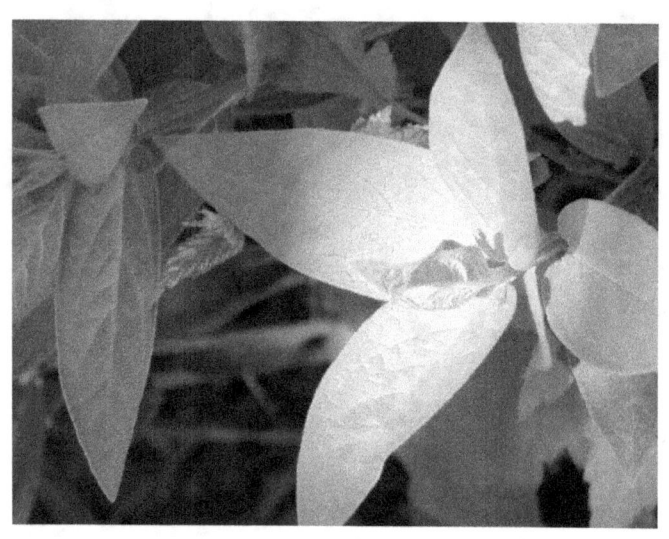

"The one who gets wisdom loves life;
the one who cherishes understanding
will soon prosper."

Proverbs 19:8 NIV

ABOUT THE AUTHOR

As a creative writer (both traditional and innovative), Deborah Johnson is a proven senior professional with integrity and a high work ethic. She has provided and will continue to provide a fresh perspective with a sound foundation in all her endeavors. A researcher, writer and speaker, Ms. Johnson has a love of the written word. She writes poetry and prose and enjoys writing opinion pieces on issues of the day.